How To Get Great Looking Skin On Face And Body

338 Tips For Maintaining Beautiful Youthful Skin

ADAM COLTON

Published by BizMove
www.bizmove.com

338 Tips For Maintaining Beautiful Youthful Skin

If you want to have healthy skin, you can reach your goal with the proper knowledge. Good skin care is the start of having beautiful skin. A solid routine requires exposure to pertinent facts about caring for skin. The tips below will take your skin care regimen to the next level.

1. Make sure your skin stays moist at all times. If your skin starts to dry out, use some moisturizer or lotion to help bring it back to life. Dry skin can be damaging and can leave your skin looking scarred. Drinking plenty of water can also help you keep your skin moist and healthy.

2. Consuming watercress regularly can actually make your skin appear less puffy, reduce inflammation and shrink pore size. You can eat watercress as part of your meal or as a snack, you can get plenty of positive effects for your skin. Your skin isn't the only thing that will benefit; watercress is rich in iron and antioxidants, which nourish your entire body.

3. Skin is the most important part of your body, and you should treat it with care at all times. Never rub your skin too hard or wear any dirty clothes, as this could have a negative chain reaction affect on the

skin on the rest of your body. Wash your clothes regularly, and treat your skin delicately.

4. Exfoliate your legs with sugar. Exfoliating your skin is very important, as it removes dead skin cells and improves blood circulation. Make a simple scrub recipe by mixing granulated sugar with a little honey or essential oil. Wash your legs with warm water and apply the sugar scrub in a circular motion. Rinse off with cold water, and moisturize immediately. Your skin will be noticeably softer and smoother.

5. To keep skin-care costs to a minimum, do your research to find the best deals. Beauty does not have to cost a fortune. There are many great resources online, including popular beauty blogs and skin-care forums, where members are more than happy to share their very best beauty bargains with you.

6. If you have terribly dry skin, you should make sure that your invest in a moisturizing cream rather than a moisturizing lotion. Lotions take longer to be absorbed into your skin, making them less effective that moisturizing creams. Keep your body moisturized the right way with creams rather than lotions.

7. One way to take care of your skin is to exfoliate longer. If you are aiming to deeply exfoliate, do not try to scrub harder as you clean your skin. Simply wipe longer because using too much pressure can actually be harmful to your skin, negating the beneficial effects of the product.

8. Smoking can significantly damage your skin in many aspects. Excessive smoking can contribute to premature wrinkling of the skin due to the lack of oxygen and nutrient flow to the blood vessels. When you smoke, you are causing your blood vessels to narrow. Collagen and elastin, are two fibers that contribute to the elasticity and strength of the skin are also severely damaged while smoking.

9. One of the most important tips to keep in mind for healthy skin is to keep yourself hydrated. If you are dehydrated, your skin will dry out, which allows bacteria to more easily penetrate the skin, as well as causing cracking and irritation. Make sure you drink 8 glasses a day.

10. To keep skin from becoming dry in the fall and winter, moisturize every single day after your bath or shower. This is the best time to take care of this part of your daily skin care routine because it takes

advantage of the moisture that has been absorbed by the skin during bathing.

11.   If you must use some sort of bleach on your skin, use a natural bleach. Even sensitive facial bleaches can sting and damage your skin. Try using a natural bleach instead. Mix milk and a bit of lemon juice. Combined, the two make a gentle bleach. Apply this to your skin.

12.   The skin on your hands can take a beating during the winter, so be sure to take good care of your hands. Cold, dry air can quickly suck the moisture from your hands which can cause them to itch and crack. Keep them well moisturized and wear cotton gloves when you go outside.

13.   Visit your local doctor or a dermatologist if you have a rash on your skin that won't go away. A skin rash can be the result of a bacterial or fungal infection or an allergic reaction to a product. Left untreated a rash can spread and cause permanent scarring on the skin.

14.   The key to getting your face really clean is to scrub your face longer. A lot of people think that you need to scrub your face harder. However, this does not help. Scrubbing your face for a longer period of time is the best way to get your face clean.

15.	If you are trying to shrink your pores, try using a mask. You can make one at home by using egg whites. You don't need any other ingredients and this can work with just one use. Egg whites tighten your skin, shrink your pores and reduce the appearance of wrinkles.

16.	Make razor burn go away by using this form of a shaving cream. Natural olive oils and typical hair conditioner are a perfect combination for an immediate shaving cream substitution. You will not only get rid of the hair, but you will also make your legs super soft and smooth.

17.	Know what type of skin you have. This can help you take care of your skin better and find products that will work for you. You should base your skin care routine on your skin type. Use products only made for your specific skin type for the best results.

18.	The beginning of the article pointed out how important proper skin care is. If you know the right way to treat your skin, you will have less chance of acne or other skin problems. Use the advice this article has given to you, and you will see your skin start looking much better.

19.   If you want to avoid getting wrinkles in your old age, try wearing sunglasses whenever you're out in bright sunlight. It's been shown that squinting so that you can see properly when in bright sunlight can be a cause of wrinkles around your eyes. A basic pair of sunglasses from the dollar store can keep you from squinting and protect you from wrinkles.

20.   This will sound obvious, but if you are looking to have better skin, you need to watch your consumption of fatty foods, particularly foods such as pork, duck and fatty red meat. Though delicious, these foods contain so much fat that you can sometimes feel it coming right out of your skin the day after you eat it. So the best way to control your skin's oil output is to get a handle on your own fat input.

21.   Always use a moisturizing cream or body lotion. Doing so will prevent many of the skin conditions caused by dry skin such as, itchiness, redness, peeling, and acne. Make sure that it is hypoallergenic as well as of the non-greasy type. This simple tip will make your life a lot easier as well as help to keep you looking fabulous.

22.   If your skin is dry, which might show as being tight and flaky, then your skin-care regime should be for dry skin. To help with this, it is advised that

you wash, tone and moisturize, both in the morning and in the evening. Cream cleansers, non-astringent toners and a good moisturizer, are recommended for this skin type.

23.   If you have terribly dry skin, you should make sure that your invest in a moisturizing cream rather than a moisturizing lotion. Lotions take longer to be absorbed into your skin, making them less effective that moisturizing creams. Keep your body moisturized the right way with creams rather than lotions.

24.   When you take a bath, you can put dry milk in the water to help your skin. If you put dry milk in the water, your body will absorb some of the richness in the milk, helping your body stay healthy and moisturized. Try this tip to keep your skin healthy and glowing.

25.   To help keep your skin looking its best, never go to bed with makeup or sunscreen on. Something that's been on your face all day is full of dirt and germs, and that can lead to breakouts. Even if you think you are too tired, be sure to wash your face before you go to sleep.

26.   If you treat your face with fruit acids, you can attain a healthier, cleaner look. By placing fruit acids

on your skin, the outer layer of dead skin is removed, causing your skin to look fresh and rejuvenated. Fruit acids also promote the generation of collagen, which helps prevent sun damage.

27.   If you have a tattoo that you no longer want, speak to a dermatologist or other skin care professional rather than trying to remove it using a commercial cream. Most tattoo removal creams are ineffective, and at best will lighten the appearance of your tattoo. Plus, the harsh chemicals in those creams may lead to a serious skin irritation.

28.   To take care of your skin--especially your face-- take the time to wash your bedding. This tip may not seem obvious at first, but it has proven critical to many acne sufferers and people with blotchy skin. We often overlook our dirty pillows and sheets. By sleeping on this dirt and oil night after night, we subject our face to added contaminants. This, in turn, may lead to poor skin.

29.   If you have extremely sensitive skin and you live in a very hot, dry climate, avoid washing your face with plain water. Many people find that in very dry weather, water washes will actually dry your skin out further. Replace it with a gentle cleanser specifically designed for sensitive skin.

30.　　If you have combination skin, that is, skin with both oily and dry areas, choose a foundation that is whipped, powder, or cream. Any of these options will do an excellent job of covering any blemishes and giving you a smooth, even tone. These types of foundation will also moisturize your skin rather than dry it out.

31.　　Exfoliating your face with a scrub will yield radiant skin over time. As you age, dead skin cells accumulate on your face, which causes you to look old. A scrub to exfoliate the cells will leave you with a better looking skin. In addition, exfoliating reduces the appearance of pores by removing oil and dirt trapped underneath the skin's surface.

32.　　For healthy skin, the first step is to keep it clean. Instead of using soaps on your face, use a face wash that is made for your skin type. Whether your face is oily, dry or combination, you can find face wash at your local drug store, department store or make-up store.

33.　　To balance your skin, try an aspirin mask. Crush a few uncoated aspirin in a teaspoon or two of warm water. Mix this into a fine paste, and apply a thin, even layer across your skin. This mask contains salcylic acid which fades acne scars and helps neutralize breakouts before they start.

34.   Supplement your intake of beta carotene. Beta carotene, or Vitamin A is a potent antioxidant and actually helps maintain the skin's defenses by beefing up its protective layer. Beta carotene also assists in the cleanup of current breakouts by making the body's natural repair process more efficient. You can amp up your vitamin A intake easily -- just eat some carrots!

35.   Your skin care regime should include a healthy diet. Fresh fruits and vegetables are packed full of nutrients that will give your complexion a boost. Foods rich in Vitamin C can aid in maintaining the skin's collagen, ensuring firmness and elasticity. Lycopene, which is found in red-colored fruits and vegetables, can help to protect the skin against damaging UV rays.

36.   If you want better skin, drop the fat-free diet. Believe it or not, your skin actually benefits from eating fats. Try adding a little more fat to your diet. Stick to healthy, unsaturated fats. Foods like olive oil, almonds and fatty fish all contain unsaturated fats that will reduce dry, itchy skin.

37.   If you have an excess amount of oil or sebum on your skin, try to use oil absorbing sheets periodically, during the day. These sheets can help

to control the oil that your body produces and limit the effect that it has on your skin. Oil helps trap bacteria, so the less oil on your skin, the better.

38.   Should you use a toner after you wash your face? The recommendations are split. A toner's job is to remove oil, makeup and dirt that is left over after cleaning your face. The fact is, a good cleaner should clean your face well enough that it does not leave behind any traces. cleanser should do this.

39.   If you are taking a bath instead of a shower, do not stay in the tub too long. The longer your body is submerged in water, the faster it will dry out, which will strip your body of the oils that it needs for optimal health. 10-15 minutes is the optimal time for a bath.

40.   When shopping for a calming aromatherapy product, you should avoid creams, lotions, or balms that contain lavender essential oils. While the fragrance may have a calming effect on your mood, the oil itself is notorious for irritating the skin and making it significantly more sensitive to the damaging effects of the sun.

41.   Baking soda is great for skin care purposes. A paste can be formed to use as an overnight pimple treatment. Baking soda can soften skin when

applied topically to rough, dry patches. Also, you can reduce some of the gunk on your scalp with this formula.

42.   To ensure that one is keeping their skin in the best condition it can be in, it is important to avoid going to artificial suntanning facilities. When one uses a fake tanning bed they are greatly increasing the damage done to their skin. Fake tanning can greatly harm a persons skin.

43.   After you shave your face or any other body part, you need to apply a moisturizing product that does not contain any alcohol or fragrances. The alcohol and scents can burn or irritate the skin on your face. You should use a soothing product that will cool and tone your skin.

44.   If you are going to get expert advice about skin care, talk directly to a dermatologist. Research shows that primary physicians are much less likely to detect abnormal skin conditions than the experts in the field of dermatology. It may cost a little extra, but if you are concerned, it will be money well spent in the end.

45.   Maximizing the amount of sleep you get each night is essential to proper skin care. If you do not get enough rest, your skin will produce an

overabundance of oil and enlarge your pores. Try going to bed 30 minutes earlier than normal and sleeping in 30 minutes later. This extra sleep will improve the overall appearance of your skin.

46. If you suffer from dry skin, it's important to use mild skin cleansers to avoid further drying your skin. Many soaps are harsher than they need to be, with antibacterial additives or irritating perfumes. Depending on what your skin can tolerate, choose either a non-foaming, non-scented body wash or one with light moisturizers.

47. If you don't really love that golden tanning look, but still would like a nice glow to your skin, it is a lot easier then you think. Just put a couple of drops of tanning lotion into your regular lotion. You won't look like you laid in the sun, but your skin will look wonderful and healthy.

48. Avoid smoking if your skin health is important to you. When you smoke, it causes the blood vessels in your face to constrict your blood flow. Wrinkles can also appear because of the facial expressions made while smoking.

49. Drink plenty of water every day. This will help your overall health as well as keep your skin moist. The skin is actually the largest organ of the body

and requires a certain amount of water to stay healthy and look its best. It is one of the easiest ways to accomplish beautiful looking skin.

50.   There are many foods that are good for your skin across the board, due to the plethora of nutrients that they contain. Turkey is a great cold cut that you can eat that is rich in zinc, iron and B vitamins. Turkey is a solid option to restore healthy cells underneath your skin.

51.   Use a face mask depending on your needs. These can usually be done once or twice a week and can make a big difference in how your skin looks. There are different masks out there for different needs and there are also masks you can make using ingredients you already have.

52.   You may think that you won't ever get to have clear and beautiful skin, but by using this advice you will be able to do just that. As this article shows, there are many ways to improve the appearance of your skin. If you use the above advice, fantastic looking skin is something you can have. Don't just keep it to yourself; when others ask about the secret of your radiant complexion, share!

53.   When you are looking for skin care products that can help you firm your skin you should look

for things that contain components like green tea, aloe-vera, Shea butter, emu oil or hyaluronic acid. Many plastic surgeons agree that these help firm your skin. Look for these or a combination of them to see the results.

54.   One of the best things you can remember for great skin is to eat the right kind of foods. A healthy balanced diet of key foods will help you to have good skin. Eat a good diet of things like nuts, seeds, eggs, and plenty of raw fruits and vegetables.

55.   Dry skin is a problem for many people, especially during the winter months. To keep skin moisturized, avoid hot water, as this will dry out your skin even further. When taking showers, or washing your face and hands, always use lukewarm water. And remember to apply moisturizer liberally, while the skin is still slightly damp.

56.   Many cosmetic companies market extra-expensive "night creams" in beautiful tiny jars. If you want the benefits of moisturizing while you sleep, save yourself some money and use a bit of the regular day cream around the skin of your eye area that you would normally use. The moisturizing benefits are the same, but your wallet will notice the difference.

57.   For beautiful, magazine-model skin, skip those extra alcoholic drinks. Research shows that drinking more than one beer, glass of wine, or cocktail per day can increase your skin's oiliness and make your pores look larger. Plus, drinking too much alcohol can dehydrate you, causing skin flakiness. Additionally, alcohol's ability to dilate blood vessels will increase redness.

58.   Get enough sleep. Your body uses the time you sleep as an opportunity to repair itself. Even everyday activities cause minor damage to your skin. If you do not get enough sleep, your skin will suffer for it. It is recommended you get a minimum of seven hours of sleep at night, though eight to ten is even better.

59.   Your skin is an organ, not just an outer shell. The skin is the largest organ in the body. Therefore, the health of your skin is important for the health of your entire body. Caring for your body will show results, both to others and to your doctor.

60.   Many people use oil-blotting sheets from the pharmacy to absorb access oil from the face during the day. If you happen to run out and need a beauty fix in a hurry, tear off a piece of a clean paper liner from the restroom. This paper has the same

absorbent properties as oil-blotting sheets you get from the store.

61.   If you are looking for matte skin, follow these simple steps. First, start off your day with a facial cleanser that lists sulfur as its main ingredient. This will keep oil at bay during the day. Second, spot-treat your oily T-zone with over-the-counter blotting sheets. Third, if you use makeup, use powder makeup instead of liquid-based foundation. These oil-bashing tips are especially effective in the summertime.

62.   Use a heavy moisturizing and nutritive product at night to hydrate and reinvigorate your skin. Your whole body uses sleep as its time for regrowth and healing. Give your skin the tools it needs to do this most effectively. Apply liberally before bed and wash off in the shower the next morning.

63.   To properly care for your skin, it is essential that you double-cleanse your face. The first cleansing should remove your makeup and sunscreen. The second wash should include a product that has rejuvenating properties to maximize the benefits to your skin. This two-step process is particularly important if you wear a lot of makeup.

64.   Are you experiencing dry skin so badly that you are considering making an appointment with the dermatologist? Before you cough up the co-pay, try these simple tips to help relieve dry skin. Instead of using soap to wash your body, use a moisturizing body wash instead, and afterward, apply a moisturizing lotion. In addition, use a humidifier in your home. It will help to relieve itchy, dry skin. If these recommendations do not remedy your dry skin, then make an appointment with your doctor.

65.   Having a hobby can help protect your skin. Stress can cause breakouts; therefore, by having a hobby, you can reduce stress.

66.   When going out with friends, avoid the temptation to drink hard liquor. Alcohol will expedite the drying out of the skin, which can ruin your appearance and hurt your health. If you do have alcohol, try to drink in moderation to reduce the negative impact on the way that you look.

67.   Treat your hands well to make them softer and less wrinkled, while brightening the nails. Use a scrub made of sugar and let it sit for a few minutes. Rinse thoroughly with warm water and moisturize with a good quality hand cream. Rub the cream thoroughly into your hands and cuticles. Then, give yourself a manicure and admire how great it looks.

68.   Eczema, acne and dry skin are conditions that can all benefit from an increased intake of essential fatty acids. Foods like cold water fish are great for your complexion, and of course, for your body in general. Try making salad dressing with flax seed oil or walnut oil to add a delicious and beneficial change to your diet, and a healthy tone to skin.

69.   In order to protect your eyes you should wear sunglasses whenever possible especially when it is very sunny and bright outside. This is when the suns UV rays are at their most dangerous. Wearing sunglasses protects the areas around your eyes from developing crows feet which is the result if continuous sun damage.

70.   If you smoke, you should try to quit smoking. Smoking damages your skin. Your skin is a very large organ and just like the rest of your body, it needs to breathe. Smoking could make your skin take on a greyish quality. No one wants skin that looks dull and lifeless. Stop smoking and let it get the clean air that it needs to look healthy and alive.

71.   Try to remove caffeine from your diet or, at the very least, try to consume less of it. Caffeine acts as a diuretic in your body. It sucks the moisture from

your skin, causing it to look less healthy. Over time, it can even decrease your skin's natural elasticity.

72.   When caring for your skin, don't forget about the areas immediately around the eyes. These areas require special moisturizing treatments, since this skin does not produce its own oil like the rest of your face. A nightly treatment with an eye area cream can keep unsightly wrinkles from forming around the eyes.

73.   Try not to overdo it with long hot baths and showers. The steamy, warm environment strips your skin of essential oils. This causes unattractive, flaky, dry skin that will have a hard time holding an moisture. Try to use warm instead of hot water and try bathing for shorter periods of time.

74.   If you have sensitive skin, don't use a harsh exfoliating scrub on your face. An exfoliating scrub that contains granules or beads is much too hard on sensitive skin. Prepare a gentle exfoliator that contains a natural ingredient such as oatmeal. Simply mix the oatmeal with a little water and apply to the skin for 20 minutes. After rinsing with warm water, your skin will be soft and have a radiant glow. People with sensitive skin should only exfoliate once a week.

75.   A good skin care tip is to avoid using soap directly on your face. Using soap is fine on your body, but using it on your face can cause the skin to dry out, which may result in a breakout. Generally, soaps should be applied below the neck.

76.   To keep your skin products from damaging your skin, you should dispose of old makeup products. Even if it doesn't have an expiration date, makeup can go bad, just like food can. In addition to this, dust and dirt can build up in makeup containers over time. For the most part, you should not keep makeup for more than 1 or 2 years.

77.   To reduce the damage that sun has done to your skin, you should apply a topical Vitamin C cream. Researchers have found that creams containing Vitamin C can decrease the effects of photodamage, and protect your skin from the sun in the future. Vitamin C can also improve the texture of your skin.

78.   Remember that moisturizing your face does only half of the job. Try to drink plenty of water because it helps in keeping your skin hydrated and looking fresh as well. Your skin is one of the largest organs in your body and also requires the most care since it is the barrier between your insides and the outside world. Drinking water rids your body and skin of

toxins, while also hydrating it; moisturizing after helps finish the job.

79.   Reduce your stress to clear up your skin. When you are overstressed, your body releases more stress hormones, such as adrenaline and cortisol. These make your skin more sensitive and prone to breakouts and cold sores. Take steps to reduce your stress, and keep your skin healthier and more radiant.

80.   When you are talking about skin care, you have to realize that there are certain parts of your body that you will usually neglect. These areas are your neck, your elbows,and heels. If you neglect these parts of your body, you will have dry patches in these areas.

81.   Fish oil can help extremely dry skin. Taking a single fish oil capsule every day will significantly improve dry skin by moisturizing from within. Not only this, but it will help to improve the texture of your hair and also strengthen brittle nails. Fish oil is particularly helpful for older skin as it maintains the production of collagen, thus decreasing the formation of wrinkles.

82.   Eliminate wrinkles, gain softer skin and have better looking nails by pampering your hand. Use a

sugar scrub for a few minutes to exfoliate. Once you wash it off, put on a heavy moisturizing cream. Rub the cream thoroughly into your hands and cuticles. Then, give yourself a manicure and admire how great it looks.

83.   Using a good, high-quality shaving gel can reduce the irritation caused by shaving and improve overall skin care. Shaving can put the skin at risk through abrasion. Many gels and foams for shaving, now include moisturizers and other ingredients, that help nourish the skin and reduce the harmful effects of using a razor.

84.   Use carrot on your skin. Grate a carrot into fine strips. Put these strips in a pot and boil them until their consistency is mushy. Rub this into the skin on your face and body. After about 15 minutes shower off. Believe it or not, this can improve the smoothness of your skin.

85.   Be cautious when shaving your skin. A good blade is exceptionally sharp, but it can damage or irritate your skin if you do not take proper precautions. Lubricate your skin with shaving cream, lotion or gel prior to shaving. Always use a clean razor for the best, smoothest shave. Do not shave against the hair, but with it so it is easier.

86.   Make sure you keep your skin clean to keep it healthy. Use a good sponge or washcloth along with warm soapy water to help remove all the built up oil from your skin. Doing this helps reduce the amount of acne you'll see. Make sure you replace your sponge or washcloth every so often to keep bacteria and germs from building up on it.

87.   To keep the skin around your eyes looking youthful, doing something as simple as just buying sunglasses can do wonders. Sunglasses don't just make you look cool. Over time, squinting into the sunlight can cause wrinkles. Putting on a pair of shades before you leave the house will prevent that from happening.

88.   One important part of skin care is to recognize your skin's lifestage, and treat it accordingly. Do you have very young skin? It will be much oilier and more elastic, responding to oil-free treatments. If your skin is over 40, you need to take a gentler approach. If you recognize that you need to deal with both oiliness and dryness, use a combination of gentle soaps and moisturizer.

89.   Your skin is porous, both absorbing things in, like sunlight and moisturizers, but also letting things out, like sweat. If you suffer from acne, it could be that your body has radicals and contaminants in it,

that normal detoxification processes like sweat, feces, and urine aren't able to remove. Purify your diet of preservatives, chemicals, and dirty foods. Stay hydrated and eat whole, preferably organic, foods, and you might see your skin clearing up within days.

90.   Believe it or not, your makeup does have an expiration date. You will need to throw out your old cosmetics at least every six to eight months, probably sooner. Bacteria and other harmful elements can grow and thrive in your makeup and that is bad for your skin.

91.   When you're moisturizing your face, smear some on your neck! Lines form there similar to the ones on foreheads, and a perfectly taken-care-of face accompanied by a crepey, lined neck still shows age! If you're prone to body acne, use your facial lotion on your chest and upper back too. It's lighter and most are listed as non-comedogenic so it won't clog your pores.

92.   If one lives in a dry area or has skin that dries out during the drier times of the year such as winter in can be crucial for them to use a lotion. Using a lotion or moisturizer will keep ones skin from painful cracking as a result of being too dry.

93.   When you are trying to moisturize your face, you should make sure that you spread lotion into your face using upward and outward motions. By doing so, you are promoting penetration of the lotion into the deeper layers of your face, promoting beautiful healthy looking skin for years to come.

94.   One of the best things you can do to care for your skin, is to check the label on the products that you buy. The less ingredients they contain, the better they will be for your skin. Try using aloe vera juice, combined with a splash of jojoba oil for a healthy glow.

95.   If you want proper skin care then you have to make sure you don't smoke. Smoking contributes to wrinkles and reduces the amount of nutrients in your body that are helpful towards healthy skin, such as vitamin A. If you do happen to smoke and can't cut the habit then try your best to reduce the amount of smoke you consume, it would be better to quit altogether but any bit helps.

96.   Dermatologists have begun to recommend a daily supplement of 1000 IU of Vitamin D3 to improve the condition of your skin. It has long been known that Vitamins A and E contribute to skin health, and now Vitamin D3 is the latest

supplement to make that list. Be sure to check with your doctor first to see what your Vitamin D levels are, and then start taking a daily supplement if needed.

97.   Try caring for your skin with a sonic skin-care brush. Especially beneficial to people with rosacea, this product helps skin maintain its normal appearance. As the brush gently exfoliates, it opens up the skin and allows other products to be more effective in calming down any irritation affecting the skin.

98.   There are two obvious factors that are detrimental to the healthiness of the facial skin. A lack of sleep will quickly take its toll leaving the skin tired and with black circles under the eyes, so ensure that you get at least seven hours sleep per day. Secondly, an over-abundance of alcohol drinking will also drain the skin of its luster and produce enlarged pores. Try to limit alcohol intake to no more than one drink per night.

99.   To take care of sensitive skin, remember this general rule of thumb; the fewer the ingredients, the more gentle the product. This is not a universal law, but it is applicable enough to use as a reliable guide. Gentle, natural products rarely have more than a handful of ingredients; harsh, synthetic products

may have a whole label-full of chemical components.

100.   Avocado is a fantastic ingredient that you can take advantage of if you have very dry skin that is hard to control. Just crush it until it's a paste and apply to the dry areas of your body. Leave it on for twenty minutes, then rinse and enjoy brighter, softer skin.

101.   Always use a high SPF sunscreen before going outside into the sunshine. The ultraviolet rays emitted from the sun can cause sunburn, premature skin aging and skin cancer. By using a sunblock on your skin, you will be able to keep youthful looking skin for longer and also reduce your risk of serious skin diseases in the future.

102.   When buying skin care products, always check the label for ingredients. A product that contains only chemicals is going to be harmful for your skin. Look for natural products that contain few ingredients. Nature contains plenty of very efficient remedies that will not harm your skin because they are not harsh like chemicals.

103.   Those wishing to improve the appearance and condition of their skin ought to enlist the help of a reputable dermatologist or professional esthetician.

Such individuals possess the expertise necessary to identify skin conditions, recommend appropriate skin care products to treat those conditions and customize a cleansing regimen suited to individual skin type.

104.   You need to remember that your lips should be included in your skin care. To have younger, fuller lips, there are steps you can take. Always use sun protection to protect them from sun damage. To keep them from looking scaly, it is important to keep them hydrated, and that is as easy as drinking enough water.

105.   Whenever you go outside, remember to use plenty of sunblock. If you fail to do this, your skin could undergo something called photo aging. The sun damages the cells in your skin and will cause your skin to prematurely age, leading to more wrinkles in your skin as you age.

106.   Diet is important in maintaining healthy skin. Care for your body and your face by taking a multi-vitamin every day. Vitamins and minerals promote healthy skin growth from within. That is the the only way to look your absolute best on the outside. A good vitamin pack will eliminate the need for additional tinctures and creams.

107.   If you are young or old and are frustrated about your skin, you must understand that the quest for healthy skin is a gradual one. To obtain healthy skin, you must follow a daily routine to keep your skin healthy. There is no one day acne miracle that will make your skin magically healthy.

108.   If you treat your face with fruit acids, you can attain a healthier, cleaner look. By placing fruit acids on your skin, the outer layer of dead skin is removed, causing your skin to look fresh and rejuvenated. Fruit acids also promote the generation of collagen, which helps prevent sun damage.

109.   If you enjoy milk, it could be bad news for your skin care. Since milk contains certain hormones, it can cause your body to trigger acne. So what can you do to get your vitamin D fix? Switch to a soy milk brand, you will still get the great flavor and all the nutrition that traditional milk provides, minus the acne.

110.   Don't pass up on using sunscreen just because it's wintertime. Your skin can be just as damaged from a bright but cold December day, as it could on the beach in August. This is even more true if there is snow on the ground, as the glare can reflect even more UV radiation onto your face.

111.   The use of salicylic acid as a facial peel can help with reducing the signs of aging, hyperpigmentation, and acne. It even minimizes the appearance of pores. Salicylic acid is an anti-flammatory that helps break down the protein bonds between several layers of skin. The use of the acid is effective in soothing and improving your skin.

112.   The skin on your baby's bottom can be kept healthier if you use a cloth diaper. Cloth diapers offer the skin an opportunity to breathe, and they are free of harsh chemicals that are found in some disposables. Cloth diapers are also often made of natural products, and therefore they feel softer on your baby's skin.

113.   If you want to banish wrinkles and other signs of aging, apply a moisturizer that contains sunscreen when you get up each morning. Sun damage is a major contributor to the appearance of fine lines and wrinkles on the face. Sunscreen in moisturizers is the best way to hydrate your face and to prevent sun damage.

114.   The skin around your eyes is extremely delicate and needs a gentle skin care routine. Rubbing and scrubbing this area can damage the tiny blood vessels under the eye, so be gentle when cleansing.

Use your ring finger to apply your under eye cream in a gentle tapping motion to boost blood circulation to this delicate part of your skin.

115.   Give your skin a break. Always remove your makeup before going to bed, using a gentle cleanser. Go makeup-free one day a week if possible. This gives your skin a chance to breathe and rejuvenate itself. If the thought of going completely barefaced doesn't appeal to you, use tinted moisturizer for a little color.

116.   When purchasing skin care products, such as moisturizers or body washes, choose products that are fragrance-free. The addition of perfumes can cause irritations, especially to sensitive skin. Less chemicals to skin care products means that their closer to a natural state.

117.   If you want to retain the moisture in your skin, try to avoid coffee as much as possible. This liquid is usually very hot and contains a lot of caffeine, which are two factors that will serve to reduce your moisture levels. Eliminate coffee from your morning regimen for clear skin.

118.   When caring for your skin, you must be sure to wash it in warm water, instead of hot or cold water. Water that is too hot or too cold, has been shown

to cause damage to the skin cells. The most common type of damage from hot water is excessive dryness, while cold water can cause wrinkles.

119.   In order to keep your skin at its healthiest and best, always wash off your makeup at night. Wearing makeup overnight can clog your pores, leading to acne breakouts and other embarrassing skin problems. A simple scrub with a pre-moistened wipe can help avoid this issue without taking too much time.

120.   People who suffer from oily skin should follow a strict skin care regime. Cleanse twice daily with a cleanser that is designed specifically for oily skin. It will remove dirt from the pores and get rid of excess oil build-up. Use a toner to remove any dirt remaining, and finally don't forget to use a light moisturizer that will help to balance the skin.

121.   It is important to purge the dead skin cells and excess debris that may form on your face while you are outside. Relaxing in a sauna, steam room or hot tub for twenty minutes can open your pores and let in oxygen, improving the way that you feel and look.

122.   Increase the effectiveness of your facial cleansing routine by using a two-step process. First, use a mild and gentle cleanser to remove cosmetics, sunscreen, and other impurities. This prepares the skin for the second step, which involves applying a soothing, hydrating moisturizer. Use gentle, upward motions to evenly spread the moisturizer over the skin.

123.   Expensive cleansers are often a waste of money. Cleansers are only on your face for a few seconds to a minute, which is not long enough for any additives to work effectively. In addition, many have harsh chemicals that can dry out or harm your skin. Instead, opt for a simple, all natural cleanser, without harsh chemicals or additives.

124.   If you have terribly dry skin, you should make sure that your invest in a moisturizing cream rather than a moisturizing lotion. Lotions take longer to be absorbed into your skin, making them less effective that moisturizing creams. Keep your body moisturized the right way with creams rather than lotions.

125.   To keep a natural, healthy glow to your skin, it's important to exfoliate. Over time, dead skin cells build up on your face, and can make your skin feel uneven or rough. Use a product that gently deep

cleans -- papaya enzyme products are good for this. Your skin will look clearer and feel softer.

126.   If you need an exfoliate for your face and wish to use an all natural method, try granulated sugar. Granulated sugar, which is very inexpensive, or sometimes free if acquired from restaurants, acts as an abrasive when massaged into the skin. It removes dead skin cells, allowing new skin cells to surface.

127.   If you have oily skin and are prone to blackheads in your T-zone, look for a nutrient-rich facial serum that contains a high proportion of Nyacinamide, which is vitamin B3, and papaya enzyme. Nyacinamide reduces the amount of oily residue on the skin's surface, and papaya enzyme exfoliates the skin and unclogs pores.

128.   Taking a pomegranate supplement may help you fight the sunshine. If you have kept track of modern skin care suggestions, you are likely terrified of the sun. It is not a entirely unreasonable feel that way. Skin care experts are right to tell you that you should always protect yourself against sun exposure. A simple pomegranate supplement boosts your skin's natural resilience to sunlight - in some cases as much as 25 percent!

129.   Be gentle to your skin. Exfoliating or scrubbing your face too often is not good at all for your skin. Gently massage your face with cleansers or facial scrubs in an upward circular motion. Skin loses its elasticity as you age and scrubbing too hard can actually cause sagging skin on your face.

130.   Don't forget to use eye cream. The skin around your eyes requires special care as it is very thin and delicate. Eye creams or gels should be an important part of your skin care regime, as applying them can slow don't the formation of crow's feet and fine lines. Also, using normal moisturizer on your eye area can cause puffy, baggy eyes.

131.   For men who are prone to skin irritation, razor bumps, or ingrown hairs, the easiest solution may be to simply grow a beard. Continually shaving over irritated skin will result in premature aging of that area. If you are extremely prone to ingrown hairs and razor bumps, you might even notice scarring over time with constant shaving. Keeping a well-trimmed beard can look just as neat without the stress on your skin.

132.   You can treat blackheads with a daily application of a mask made of lime juice and groundnut oil. Use a teaspoon each of the two liquids. Wash your face then apply the mask. Leave it on for five

minutes then rinse your face thoroughly with warm water. Follow up with cold water and a natural toner of white vinegar or witch hazel.

133.   You will want to pick the type of soap you use very carefully. Opt for something that is all natural and free from scents. Follow up with a toner and moisturizer for sensitive skin.

134.   If you want better skin, drop the fat-free diet. Believe it or not, your skin actually benefits from eating fats. Try adding a little more fat to your diet. Stick to healthy, unsaturated fats. Foods like olive oil, almonds and fatty fish all contain unsaturated fats that will reduce dry, itchy skin.

135.   Once in a while, take the time to use a facial mask. Facial masks will tighten the skin and draw out small impurities as they dry. You can spend a lot of money on masks, or you can make your own from beaten egg whites. Just put on beaten egg white (avoiding eye area), wait for it to dry and wash off gently with warm water. Your skin will feel fresh and brand new.

136.   Vitamin E is among the best vitamins that you can take to enhance the quality of your skin. This vitamin aids in soothing the acne that you have, by smoothing the surface of your skin to maximize

comfort. Also, vitamin E helps to fade the scars that you get from acne.

137.   If you have sensitive, easily irritated skin, avoid skincare products that claim to create a tingling or plumping effect. While many consumers view these products as innovative or futuristic, these sensations are actually indicative of irritation and inflammation of the skin. Rather than risk redness or breakouts, stick with tried-and-true skincare products.

138.   When you start to wear eye cream at night, be sure you know how to apply it properly. Do not roughly rub it on your skin. Instead, line a few dots of the cream under your eyes and on the eye lids. Gently pat the area around your eyes with the pads of your fingers until the cream blends in with your skin.

139.   When you are looking for skincare products, go for simple. The more simple the formula, the better results you will get. This is especially true for your wallet. Oftentimes, products will say they are two different things when, in fact, they are the same product with a minimal variation.

140.   In the cold months you should use a humidifier, especially if you have central heat. Central heating systems push out hot, dry air through out the

building. This air can damage and dry out your skin. Using a humidifier can add moisture in the air, help you breathe better, and keep your skin from drying out.

141.   To keep your skin looking healthy and smooth, be sure to shave carefully. A gel or cream applied before shaving, will ensure that the razor glides smoothly, rather than roughing up the skin. To avoid in-grown hairs, always shave in the direction that the hair is growing, not against it.

142.   You can give yourself a very beneficial facial massage. A facial massage helps your skin absorb moisturizers and oils much faster. Dispense a small amount of oil or moisturizer into your hands. Work your moisturizer or oil into your skin around your face in a circular motion, making sure to avoid the eyes.

143.   If you would like the appearance of smoother, softer feet, then at bedtime, grab a bottle of olive oil from your kitchen cabinet and rub on a generous amount. Afterwards, throw on a pair of cotton socks on your feet and sleep with them on overnight. It may not be very attractive to wear cotton socks to bed, but you will reap the benefits with softer, smoother feet in the morning.

144.   To help your skin look its best, consider cutting back on the amount of milk you drink. Studies have shown that individuals who drink large quantities of milk experience more break-outs. Milk contains hormones, which can exacerbate skin problems. Try using soy milk as an alternative to cow's milk.

145.   Any skin care routine can be made more effective with the addition of adequate restful sleep every night. Your overall skin quality is adversely affected by the stress to your system caused by lack of sleep. Getting a good night's sleep is the one highly effective beauty treatment for your skin that is absolutely free.

146.   Healthy skin care begins by protecting yourself from the harmful effects of the sun. Continual exposure to the sun damages skin. There are several simple ways to protect skin from danger. Apply sunscreen daily and more frequently when spending time outdoors. Wear protective clothing or special apparel with UVA blockage built in.

147.   Learn to determine whether a reaction is a matter of sensitive skin or an actual allergy. While both conditions can have similar symptoms like redness, burning, or swelling, the proper treatment for each one is different. Consult a comprehensive online dermatological resource like dermatlas.org,

which contains images and information to help you determine whether you are experiencing an allergy or just sensitivity.

148.   Harsh chemotherapy and radiation treatments can wreak havoc on any skin type. Skin becomes infinitely more sensitive, so avoid conditions which are hot and humid as these tend to exacerbate the problem and result in excessive tenderness and redness. This includes saunas and spas, Jacuzzis, and even long, hot baths or showers.

149.   Avoid alcohol if you can. Alcohol can make you dehydrated, which will make your skin look bad. If you must drink alcohol, make sure you drink enough water to rehydrate your skin the next day. Staying hydrated makes your skin look great and helps to keep your complexion glowing and clear.

150.   Eat a balanced diet in order to keep your skin looking it's youngest. Work from the inside of your body and eat foods that are healthy. Yellow and orange vegetables are good for your skin because they contain beta carotene which is the best for your skin because they contain vitamin A.

151.   To protect your skin, you should wear sunscreen every time you plan to spend time outdoors. Sun exposure can damage your skin, leading to freckles,

age spots, wrinkles, dry skin and possibly even skin cancer. Choose a sunscreen with a high SPF so that you can be sure it will provide adequate protection.

152.   Maintain healthy skin by using a moisturizing soap. Regular soap can dry out your skin, which leads to less elasticity, wrinkles, and can cause irritated skin to become dry and flaky. If your skin becomes irritated then it is likely you will scratch at it, which can then lead to infection.

153.   Apple cider vinegar is great for acne. The cider will replenish moisture where acne has dried out your skin. Use it during the day since the smell of the vinegar is strong. You don't need it on your sheets.

154.   Sometimes colorless bumps, called keratosis pilaris, can form on the back of your arms. To help prevent these from forming, use a lotion that contains lactic acid twice a day. Every time you take a shower, make sure that you scrub the affected area with a loofa for at least thirty seconds. These steps help unclog the pores and smooth the bumps.

155.   Taking care of your skin is easy if you follow three simple steps. Cleansing is the first step, and you should choose a cleanser made for your skin type. Next is to use a toner, which tends to shrink

pores and removes any cleanser remaining on your face. The third step is to moisturize, but be sure to seal in the moisture, apply it before the toner is completely dry.

156.   Your skin needs to be protected from UVA and UVB rays to keep it in the best possible condition and protected from sun damage. You should always opt for a broad spectrum coverage formula for the best protection. One with at least an SPF of 15 is recommended and should be applied every two hours. Remember, sun screen should not be kept longer than a year.

157.   Looking for more beautiful skin? Make sure you get plenty of sleep each night. When you sleep, your body repairs and heals the damage to your skin brought on by stress throughout the day. Not getting at least 7 hours of sleep can leave your skin looking uneven and pale. Getting a good night's sleep will have your skin looking radiant and healthy.

158.   When shopping for sunblocks, look for products that contain titanium dioxide or zinc oxide, as these two ingredients form a physical barrier and not just a chemical one. Also, be aware of the differences in coverage implied by the different SPF ratings. Even an SPF 50 product

blocks only 98% of UV rays; in other words, no product blocks absolutely everything.

159.   Another great way to prevent your skin from looking dead and lifeless is to use tea tree oil to revitalize your skin. This fine natural product has been proven to prevent and treat a variety of skin problems. Tree tea oil is a great tool to get your skin on the right track today.

160.   One of the most overlooked parts of your face, when it comes to skin care tips is your lips. Your lips play a vital role throughout your entire skin care agenda and have some of the thinnest skin on your entire body. It is important that you take extra steps to ensure that this delicate skin remains safe and well taken care of.

161.   Smoking can significantly damage your skin in many aspects. Excessive smoking can contribute to premature wrinkling of the skin due to the lack of oxygen and nutrient flow to the blood vessels. When you smoke, you are causing your blood vessels to narrow. Collagen and elastin, are two fibers that contribute to the elasticity and strength of the skin are also severely damaged while smoking.

162.   Managing stress is an important element in taking care of your skin. A lot of skin related conditions, such as acne and breakouts, can be caused by too much stress. It is important to establish realistic goals, manage your daily activities, and take care of your health. Take some time out to relax and enjoy yourself, as a result your skin will look much better.

163.   When considering skin care products as you age, there may be no need to avoid products containing oils. Your skin produces less natural oils as you age. Moisturizers containing oil are unlikely to cause breakouts and can help keep your skin smooth and healthy by replenishing the oils that can protect skin.

164.   An important tip about skin care for your baby is to know how to cure a condition known as prickly heat. This is important to know so that you can end the discomfort for your baby. This can be prevented and cured by making sure your baby is kept in a cool and dry area with loose fitting clothes.

165.   A great skin care tip is to be sure you get a good amount of sleep every night. A lack of sleep can increase your pores and oil production. You should aim to get seven to eight hours every night. Sleep is

an important component of overall health, so it should not be ignored.

166.   An important way to protect your skin is not to smoke. Smoking makes your skin appear older and wrinkled by depriving your outer layer of skin oxygen, effectively killing it. If you smoke and are concerned about taking care of your skin, your best course of action is to quit.

167.   To take care of your skin as well as the rest of your health, it is vital to drink plenty of water. Drinking enough water helps your skin to better retain moisture. It also helps to increase your overall health, which will show in the quality and healthfulness of your skin.

168.   Overuse of makeup can cause acne issues to worsen. Most varieties of cosmetics, including powders, concealers and foundations, have pore-clogging potential. This can make the acne you suffer with even worse. If you choose to apply makeup over your acne, you are making way for infection. It is a good idea to avoid wearing makeup, whenever possible, until your acne goes away. Also, try not to use concealers or heavy toners to hide them.

169.   There is no "end-all cure" for acne breakouts.,
There are only treatments and maintenance that can
be applied daily to either reduce or possibly
eliminate the breakouts for long periods of time.
Discussing your situation with a dermatologist can
help you find a treatment or maintenance routine
for your needs to have healthier skin.

170.   Egg whites are effective in reducing the redness
of acne scarring. Separate the white from the yolk,
and whip it until it stiffens up slightly. Liberally
apply all over your face, and allow it to harden. This
should take about 15 minutes. After washing it off,
you will notice that it has eased the redness. Not
only that, egg whites help to tighten up your pores,
giving your skin a much smoother look.

171.   For extra soft and moisturized skin, spritz your
body and face with a water bottle before
moisturizing your skin with alcohol-free lotion.
Make sure you don't use hard water. Along with its
normal moisturizing abilities, the lotion also works
to lock the water in to keep your skin exceptionally
soft and youthful looking.

172.   If you want to add nutrients to your skin, then
use a facial serum over a moisturizer because a
serum allows nutrients to get deeper into the layers
of skin. If you use a moisturizer, it does not

penetrate as deeply as serums can, but is designed to add moisture to hydrate your skin.

173.   When you are putting on hand cream, don't forget to put a bit of lotion on your elbows. This easy step can help your elbows to look better and feel softer. A little bit of lotion goes a long way on the elbows. Do not overlook this part of your body, because elbows need love, too.

174.   Try using apricot oil or almond oil as a make up remover for natural skin care. It will not clog your pores and is an effective and cost efficient product. It also acts as a moisturizer. It is not a harsh chemical and works just as well as any over-the-counter make up remover.

175.   Knowing your skin type is a essential for great skin care. If you have sensitive skin, you will want to avoid things such as harsh facial peels. If you have dry skin, you'll want to focus more on moisturizing.

176.   Take care of your hands especially during the winter. The cold weather can dry out and crack the thin skin on your hands. Wear gloves when going outside and invest in a pair that will keep you nice and warm. To reverse dryness, use a heavy

moisturizer and wear cotton gloves to bed to allow the healing to begin.

177.   Who doesn't want to have soft and glowing skin? If you want to stay looking young, healthy, and radient, make sure that you always wear sunscreen! Many face creams now include sunscreen in their formulas, and at just a few bucks a bottle, it's much cheaper than any procedure done at a dermatologist!

178.   You must be extremely careful when shaving. A good blade is exceptionally sharp, but it can damage or irritate your skin if you do not take proper precautions. Also, add a layer of protection and lubrication with shaving cream, lotion or gel. A clean razor means a better shave. Shave with hair and not against it if you want to make it easier.

179.   An excellent ingredient to help care for dry skin is an avocado. Put the avacado on your face after crushing it up. Leave it on for twenty minutes, then rinse and enjoy brighter, softer skin.

180.   To prevent dirt from accumulating in your pores, you should make sure to wash your face in warm water and then splash your face with cool water. Washing with warm water opens up your pores, which allows accumulated dirt to be removed

more easily. However, if our pores remain open, they would be more prone to getting dirt back in them. On the other hand, finishing your face wash routine with cool water, helps to close your pores back up and keep your skin clean and healthy.

181.   Exfoliation plays a big role in helping you to maintain the health of your skin. Each day, dead skin cells remain on our face and body. By exfoliating your skin regularly, you remove these dead skin cells, helping to brighten your complexion and give you a more youthful, healthy appearance.

182.   Before you shave your sensitive skin, examine it to become aware of any bumps, nicks or imperfections. By being familiar with the landscape, you can avoid the pain and irritation of slicing an uneven patch of skin. Gently shave around these areas and moisturize your sensitive skin with healing aloe gel to help soothe and smooth them.

183.   If you have an excess amount of oil or sebum on your skin, try to use oil absorbing sheets periodically, during the day. These sheets can help to control the oil that your body produces and limit the effect that it has on your skin. Oil helps trap bacteria, so the less oil on your skin, the better.

184.   Sunscreen is best applied with makeup sponges. Not only does applying sunscreen with a sponge let you avoid the greasy texture of the lotion, it also helps you spread it more evenly. Dab the sunscreen onto your skin with a sponge to help it get into the skin and ensure it all gets in.

185.   Don't forget to moisturize your hands. Skin on the hands has fewer oil glands and is thinner than the skin on most parts of the human body. As a result, hands can often become itchy, dry and cracked during the winter months or when constantly exposed to water. To protect your hands, regularly apply liberal amounts of high quality moisturizer and always wear cotton gloves under rubber gloves when washing up.

186.   IF you have a oily skin type, do not think you do not have to moisturize. Once you rinse off your face, put on a moisturizer. While you may be unsure of its benefits, a good moisturizer will help with oil production. If your oily skin gets irritated, it can produce even more oil.

187.   If you have dry skin, and need an intense, or deep moisturizing treatment, use vitamin E or aloe vera oil. You can find it as a liquid, or you can just break open a capsule and apply directly to your face.

This works great on under eye areas where sagging and wrinkles appear first.

188.   To get better looking skin naturally, you should drink lots of water. While moisturizers replenish your skin from the outside, water can hydrate your skin from the inside, leaving you with a natural glow. Water also improves your circulation, and drinking plenty of it can keep you from looking overly pale or washed out.

189.   The secret to great skin is great skin care. This means that not only should your skin be cleaned and moisturized correctly for your skin type, you should also protect your skin with sun screen. This prevents serious damage and aging that the sun can cause over time. A good sun screen or make up with SPF in it can be very beneficial.

190.   Are you experiencing dry skin so badly that you are considering making an appointment with the dermatologist? Before you cough up the co-pay, try these simple tips to help relieve dry skin. Instead of using soap to wash your body, use a moisturizing body wash instead, and afterward, apply a moisturizing lotion. In addition, use a humidifier in your home. It will help to relieve itchy, dry skin. If these recommendations do not remedy your dry skin, then make an appointment with your doctor.

191.   If you want to reduce the irritation on any part of your skin, invest in tea tree oil. Use three parts tea tree oil and one part water, to create a mixture that you can use to exfoliate the outer layer of your face. This will also help to reduce irritation and create a beautiful palette for attacking your day in style.

192.   To start out your day and improve the look of your skin, try to drink a lot of water or a tasty fruit smoothie. A fruit smoothie is one of the most delicious and refreshing things that you can have, also maintaining the vitamins that you need during the day.

193.   One of the best ways to attain healthy skin is to become a vegetarian or minimize your meat intake daily. This decision will help to increase the amount of fruits and vegetables that are in your diet by default, illuminating your skin and liberating your body from the toxins that yield poor skin.

194.   Looking for a great skin care cleanser to help you fight acne that you can make at home? Try heating lemon juice until warm, do not boil the juice as it will lose it's properties. Whip two egg whites into the warm lemon juice to create a foamy wash.

Promptly store the rest of the mixture in the refrigerator.

195.   Avoid tanning machines if you can. The artificial rays from a tanning bed can accelerate skin aging and even lead to cancer. If you must use them, do it infrequently. Sunless tanning lotion is a viable option, but remember to check the label on the bottle for dangerous or harmful chemicals.

196.   An important tip to consider when concerning acne is to be sure that you drink enough water. This is important because it is a healthy way to keep your skin from drying out. If you do not have enough water in your body to keep your skin moist then your body will produce more oil, increasing your chances of acne.

197.   Taking care of your skin is a great way to keep looking your best. Doing activities that help lower your stress level is one of the best ways to keep your skin healthy and beautiful. Taking a walk outside, reading, taking a relaxing bath and doing some yoga are one a few of the many different ways to help keep you stress free and your skin healthy.

198.   One of the obvious points of skin care is the daily cleansing of your face and pores. If you resist this regular routine, your pores can build up and

you will notice annoying blackheads beginning to appear. Simply rinsing them out nightly with warm soap and water is just enough to get the job done.

199.   For great skin care after you wash your face correctly you should use a exfoliant. Find the correct one for your skin type and try to get a granular one. That way it can help scrub off your dead skin cells and help to smooth the rough areas on your face which ca help your lotion work better.

200.   When using a facial scrub to exfoliate your skin, be careful about the products you use. Facial scrubs contain grains which help to loosen dead and dry skin. Be sure to choose a scrub with small, fine grains. The larger ones can badly damage your skin, irritating it and causing small abrasions.

201.   In order to have healthy, clean skin, you must stay hydrated. That means drinking around 8 cups of water every day. If you don't drink enough water, your face will become oily which will lead to pimples, acne, and other unpleasant things. Not only will you look better by staying hydrated, but you'll feel better too!

202.   Fast food is one of the worst things that you can consume during the course of the day for your skin. Usually, this type of food is filled with fat and oil

due to the poor quality and method of cooking. At night, try not to give into your cravings for fast food, if you desire healthy skin.

203.   When it's cold outside, be sure to protect your hands with gloves. The skin on your hands is thin, and it can easily get irritated and crack. Wearing gloves during this time can ensure your hands are safe and well hydrated.

204.   To soothe red and irritating skin, try drinking green tea. Green tea has natural anti-inflammatory properties that can calm an inflamed complexion. The beverage also contains epigallocatechin gallate, which naturally boosts your skin's level of collagen production. This leaves your skin looking healthier, and increases its ability to protect itself from irritants.

205.   The use of salicylic acid as a facial peel can help with reducing the signs of aging, hyperpigmentation, and acne. It even minimizes the appearance of pores. Salicylic acid is an anti-flammatory that helps break down the protein bonds between several layers of skin. The use of the acid is effective in soothing and improving your skin.

206.   Different people have different types of skin. To determine the best skin care method for yourself, you should determine what skin type you have. There are four skin types that people generally have. The types are normal skin, oily skin, dry skin, and combination skin. Knowing which skin types is yours will help you choose products and remedies that are best suited for enhancing your skin.

207.   Certain types of tea can be great for your skin. According to research, green tea and black tea have a lot of benefits for your skin. The teas contain protective items, such as EGCG, that may help prevent some skin cancers and it can also slow down the breakdown of collagen.

208.   If you wear powder during the course of the day, eliminate this as much as possible. Power can seep into the wrinkles of your skin and clog your pores, producing blemishes and uneven skin. Instead, use a moisturizer or oil absorbing sheets to maintain a dry, clean look to your face.

209.   When removing makeup and excess grime from your face at the end of the day, it is advisable to do this in a two step process. First, use a gentle cleanser to remove makeup and sunscreen products. Next, use a secondary cleanser designed to soothe and replenish the now clean skin. As with any facial

skin regime, ensure that all hand strokes are in an upward motion from the neck up.

210.   Getting enough sleep is a great way to have your skin looking good. Try to get in at least 8 hours a night. It will help your skin and face bring out that healthy shine. There is a reason why it's called beauty rest. So next time you go to bed, know that you are doing a wonderful thing for your skin.

211.   Keeping the skin on your hands healthy is just as important as keeping your facial skin healthy. Having rough hands can actually cause an infection or fungus to grow. When doing chores or manual labor, wear rubber gloves. At nighttime, gently rub lotion all over your hands, even rubbing into the skin surrounding your nails. Remove any excess lotion.

212.   Use a moisturizer on your child two times a day if they have dry skin. Do not use moisturizers that contain any fragrances, because these are specifically meant for adult skin. Visit a medical professional if the problem does not go away.

213.   Acne and other skin eruptions should never be treated by squeezing, popping or other direct contact. Not only do such actions spread infectious bacteria to other vulnerable skin areas, but the

fingers also transfer dirt and oil to the affected areas. Other treatments are far more reliable and safe for resolving acne successfully.

214.   If you enjoy the relaxing effects of a calming fragrance during your bathing ritual, try lighting candles or fragrance burners rather than using scented bath products. Most skincare products for the bath are heavily laden with excessive dyes and fragrances. These ingredients, while pleasantly scented, are known to trigger allergic reactions and to irritate sensitive skin.

215.   Once in a while, take the time to use a facial mask. Facial masks will tighten the skin and draw out small impurities as they dry. You can spend a lot of money on masks, or you can make your own from beaten egg whites. Just put on beaten egg white (avoiding eye area), wait for it to dry and wash off gently with warm water. Your skin will feel fresh and brand new.

216.   To prevent breakouts of acne, try using facial care products that come in a spray-on applicator. This will keep you from transferring bacteria, oils and potentially irritating substances from your hands to your face while applying things like sunscreen or moisturizer. Having a more bacteria-

free face can in turn reduce your chances of developing pimples.

217.   Whether your skin tone is light or dark, always use sunscreen on sunny days. Not only does over-exposure to sunlight cause skin cancer, it also ages your skin much faster. If you have an especially light complexion, avoid tanning too much. When you reduce your skin's exposure to the sun, you will reduce years to your appearance.

218.   Although it may seem counter-intuitive, immersing dry skin in water for extended periods of time may actually have a dehydrating effect. This is especially true of prolonged exposure to hot or warm water, like that found in a bath or shower. Instead, use a water soluble moisturizer and wash your face with tepid, not hot, water.

219.   Use jasmine oil on your skin. Jasmine oil soothes your skin and contains many antioxidants that prevent your skin from aging too fast. Apply a little bit of oil every morning to condition your skin and make it look bright and healthy. Do not use any kind of oil if your face easily breaks out.

220.   If you have dry skin, try applying a few drops of jojoba oil. This oil is very similar to the oil on your skin. It is easily absorbed, and it does not clog

pores. Jojoba does not evaporate quickly like water-based moisturizers, so it will help your skin retain moisture all day. A little bit goes a long way.

221. Use a natural facial mask every other week. A facial mask can help in eliminating dead, flaky skin from your face. It deep cleans your face of impurities that can clog your pores and cause acne. It can also improve the texture of your skin while giving a boost to the circulation.

222. Drinking plenty of water every day is important, as it keeps your skin smooth, moist, and soft. Mineral water is even better for your skin, though it can cost more money than some people like to spend. Try to drink at least sixty-four ounces of water every day for the best results.

223. A great skin care tip is to be aware of certain skin care myths. A common myth is that drinking a lot of water will give you great looking, healthy skin. The truth is, the amount of water a person drinks has little to no impact on how healthy their skin is.

224. Don't go to the tanning salon or tan yourself in the sun. It is bad for your skin, and can cause your skin to age prematurely. Excessive tanning can even lead to skin cancer. Instead, play it safe and use a bronzing lotion that you can safely apply to your

skin and can give you the appearance of a sun kissed tan.

225.   Better skin care with chocolate works well. While some characteristics of chocolate may be unpleasant, you can certainly enjoy the positive effects that it has on your skin. Powered with flavonoids, chocolate supplements your skin with more of those delightful chemicals that help block out the effects of harmful UV light.

226.   Always test out skin care products before you apply them to your face. Oftentimes people apply them only to find out later that they are heavily allergic to something. Take a small sample and put some of the product on a small area of your face or the back of your wrist for testing. If you're allergic to something, you will find out within minutes as your skin turns red or itches.

227.   Toner is one of the best things that you can use on your skin. A great toner will help to get rid of the impurities on your skin and even out the look of your face. Apply toner after you wash your face in the shower and follow with a top quality moisturizer with SPF.

228.   Cleanse your skin 1-2 times every day with lukewarm water for healthy skin. Regular cleansing

removes dirt and other damaging residues from your skin. If you are outside during the day, this is especially important as you are exposed to more pollutants and dust. It is always best to make sure to cleanse with lukewarm water because both hot and cold water damage your skin.

229.   Sagging skin and wrinkles can be caused by lack of sleep and exercise. These are important steps to good physical health and your skin's health. The lack of sleep and exercise can lead to becoming over stressed and can make you appear much older than what you really are.

230.   If you are planning to purchase makeup over the counter, make sure it is noncomedo If you have severely dry skin on your hands, it can and should be treated with an antibiotic cream, like you would use on cuts and scrapes. In many cases, extremely dry skin crack open and bleeds. If these cuts are ignored they can become worse - leading to scarring or even an infection. Care for them early by applying an antibiotic cream before applying moisturizer.

231.   A skin care tip for rosacea sufferers is to make liberal use of one of the new sonic skin brushes currently on the market. Though such tools can be relatively expensive, their exfoliating action makes

facial skin more receptive to topical treatments that help minimize the redness associated with the condition.

232.   Hair removal often comes with an unwanted result: ingrown hairs. After you wax or shave, exfoliate the area with a loofa or an over-the-counter scrub each time you take a shower. Make sure to scrub the skin for at least thirty seconds. Moisturize with aloe vera gel afterward. This will prevent ingrown hairs from forming.

233.   If you have dry and sore feet, you can cure and prevent this condition, by applying a silicone-based lubricant on your feet every morning. This will moisturize your feet and form a protective coat around your skin. You should probably use lubricant every time you wear brand new shoes, especially if you are going to wear them bare feet.

234.   To subtract years of age from your face, don't neglect your neck. A smooth and supple facial complexion is certainly envied, but not if it sits atop a less-than-smooth or sagging neck. You will look like you are wearing a mask or feel the need to wear turtleneck sweaters year-long, unless you treat that delicate neck skin as carefully as you treat your face. Slather moisturizer on your neck at night to create the perfect pedestal for your pretty face.

235.   Dry skin sufferers whose condition has become painful should stop using all harsh astringents, facial masks or peels. Such products have the propensity to strip important oils from the skin's surface, exacerbating existing problems. Rather, such individuals should choose mild, alcohol-free cleansers formulated to provide extra hydration.

236.   Don't go to the tanning salon or tan yourself in the sun. It is bad for your skin, and can cause your skin to age prematurely. Excessive tanning can even lead to skin cancer. Instead, play it safe and use a bronzing lotion that you can safely apply to your skin and can give you the appearance of a sun kissed tan.

237.   Change your moisturizer with the seasons. To keep your skin from drying out in the winter, switch from a light water-based moisturizer to a heavier oil-based one. The best oils for the face are avocado, primrose, almond, or mineral oil as these won't clog your pores. Avoid using shea butter on your face.

238.   If you are suffering from redness of the skin, avoid heat when you can, both internally and externally. Heading to the sauna will leave you with quite the red face. The heat will break capillaries in

the skin which is what causes the appearance of redness. Spicy hot foods like peppers will also have the same affect.

239.   Take a consultation appointment with a dermatologist to learn more about your skin. Everyone's skin is different and a product that works on your best friend may do nothing for you. A consultation will allow you to find out what kind of skin you have and what type of products you should be seeking out.

240.   For optimal cleansing and pampering of your precious skin you should always use the very best water. These waters will be free of excess minerals and chemicals and will leave your skin residue free. The best waters to use are bottled varieties, filtered types, mineral free, and freshly melted snow.

241.   To help fight against skin cancer while benefiting from healing properties of the sun, be sure to use an oil-free sunscreen. Tanning or using a sun lamp may help hide your acne, yet you don't want to end up with the long-term effects of the sun's radiation. It is healthy for your skin to spend at least 15 minutes outside in direct sunlight. Just do not over do it!

242.   Who doesn't want to have soft and glowing skin? If you want to stay looking young, healthy, and radient, make sure that you always wear sunscreen! Many face creams now include sunscreen in their formulas, and at just a few bucks a bottle, it's much cheaper than any procedure done at a dermatologist!

243.   Simply being able to pronounce all the ingredients in your face and body products means that you'll be more likely to spot ingredients that irritate your skin. A switch to natural products means your money goes a longer way, and your skin will only absorb natural products. Remember, what you put it in is what you get out of something, and your skin is the largest organ on your body.

244.   You can treat blackheads with a daily application of a mask made of lime juice and groundnut oil. Use a teaspoon each of the two liquids. Wash your face then apply the mask. Leave it on for five minutes then rinse your face thoroughly with warm water. Follow up with cold water and a natural toner of white vinegar or witch hazel. genic. This type of makeup will not clog your pores and is safe to use every single day. Avoiding the types of products that will do harm to your skin is important in your skin care regimen.

245.   If you have severely dry skin on your hands, it can and should be treated with an antibiotic cream, like you would use on cuts and scrapes. In many cases, extremely dry skin crack open and bleeds. If these cuts are ignored they can become worse - leading to scarring or even an infection. Care for them early by applying an antibiotic cream before applying moisturizer.

246.   A skin care tip for rosacea sufferers is to make liberal use of one of the new sonic skin brushes currently on the market. Though such tools can be relatively expensive, their exfoliating action makes facial skin more receptive to topical treatments that help minimize the redness associated with the condition.

247.   Hair removal often comes with an unwanted result: ingrown hairs. After you wax or shave, exfoliate the area with a loofa or an over-the-counter scrub each time you take a shower. Make sure to scrub the skin for at least thirty seconds. Moisturize with aloe vera gel afterward. This will prevent ingrown hairs from forming.

248.   If you have dry and sore feet, you can cure and prevent this condition, by applying a silicone-based lubricant on your feet every morning. This will moisturize your feet and form a protective coat

around your skin. You should probably use lubricant every time you wear brand new shoes, especially if you are going to wear them bare feet.

249.   To subtract years of age from your face, don't neglect your neck. A smooth and supple facial complexion is certainly envied, but not if it sits atop a less-than-smooth or sagging neck. You will look like you are wearing a mask or feel the need to wear turtleneck sweaters year-long, unless you treat that delicate neck skin as carefully as you treat your face. Slather moisturizer on your neck at night to create the perfect pedestal for your pretty face.

250.   Dry skin sufferers whose condition has become painful should stop using all harsh astringents, facial masks or peels. Such products have the propensity to strip important oils from the skin's surface, exacerbating existing problems. Rather, such individuals should choose mild, alcohol-free cleansers formulated to provide extra hydration.

251.   Don't go to the tanning salon or tan yourself in the sun. It is bad for your skin, and can cause your skin to age prematurely. Excessive tanning can even lead to skin cancer. Instead, play it safe and use a bronzing lotion that you can safely apply to your skin and can give you the appearance of a sun kissed tan.

252. Change your moisturizer with the seasons. To
      keep your skin from drying out in the winter, switch
      from a light water-based moisturizer to a heavier
      oil-based one. The best oils for the face are
      avocado, primrose, almond, or mineral oil as these
      won't clog your pores. Avoid using shea butter on
      your face.

253. If you are suffering from redness of the skin,
      avoid heat when you can, both internally and
      externally. Heading to the sauna will leave you with
      quite the red face. The heat will break capillaries in
      the skin which is what causes the appearance of
      redness. Spicy hot foods like peppers will also have
      the same affect.

254. Take a consultation appointment with a
      dermatologist to learn more about your skin.
      Everyone's skin is different and a product that
      works on your best friend may do nothing for you.
      A consultation will allow you to find out what kind
      of skin you have and what type of products you
      should be seeking out.

255. For optimal cleansing and pampering of your
      precious skin you should always use the very best
      water. These waters will be free of excess minerals
      and chemicals and will leave your skin residue free.

The best waters to use are bottled varieties, filtered types, mineral free, and freshly melted snow.

256.   To help fight against skin cancer while benefiting from healing properties of the sun, be sure to use an oil-free sunscreen. Tanning or using a sun lamp may help hide your acne, yet you don't want to end up with the long-term effects of the sun's radiation. It is healthy for your skin to spend at least 15 minutes outside in direct sunlight. Just do not over do it!

257.   Who doesn't want to have soft and glowing skin? If you want to stay looking young, healthy, and radient, make sure that you always wear sunscreen! Many face creams now include sunscreen in their formulas, and at just a few bucks a bottle, it's much cheaper than any procedure done at a dermatologist!

258.   Simply being able to pronounce all the ingredients in your face and body products means that you'll be more likely to spot ingredients that irritate your skin. A switch to natural products means your money goes a longer way, and your skin will only absorb natural products. Remember, what you put it in is what you get out of something, and your skin is the largest organ on your body.

259.   You can treat blackheads with a daily application of a mask made of lime juice and groundnut oil. Use a teaspoon each of the two liquids. Wash your face then apply the mask. Leave it on for five minutes then rinse your face thoroughly with warm water. Follow up with cold water and a natural toner of white vinegar or witch hazel.

260.   Have healthier skin by not smoking. Not only is smoking hazardous to your heath, but it can destroy your skin as well by causing it to wrinkle. What the smoke does is restrict blood flow in the blood vessels in your face, depleting your skin of much needed oxygen and nutrients. This also depletes the collagen in your skin, causing it to sag and wrinkle.

261.   If you have sensitive skin, avoid using cosmetics that are not natural or hypoallergenic. Many popular makeup brands contain harsh irritants, fragrances and other chemicals that can completely irritate your skin. Stick to all-natural cosmetics free of these ingredients and make sure not to mix too many brands as this can also cause a reaction.

262.   Finding the perfect foundation at a drugstore can be a tricky proposition. If you want to be sure the shade you're choosing looks as close as possible to your skin, you need to do two things. First, put a dab of the tester on the back of your hand, where

the skin will match your facial skin. Secondly, if possible, try to move to where you can examine your hand in natural light. Natural light will give you the best possible idea of how your foundation will look on your face out in the real world.

263.   If you have oily skin, don't use moisturizer. This is the equivalent of using butter and mayonnaise on a sandwich: one is oily enough. On the other hand, you may be oily all over with a few dry areas, generally near the eyes or on the cheeks back near your ears. In that case, apply moisturizer only to the dry areas of your face.

264.   One of the best things you can do to care for your skin, is to apply a lip balm with UV protection. Your lips contain extremely thin skin, which means they need extra protection from the sun. The use of lip balm will keep them from getting chapped and help prevent skin cancer from forming.

265.   Prevent the sun from ruining the work you have put into skin care. Everyone knows that harmful UV rays can damage and destroy your skin. One of the easiest ways to avoid this is by applying sunscreen. As this can sweat off as your active, it can help to apply a thin layer of UV protection, followed by a mix of minerals that naturally block out UV light.

266. Use a shaving gel with aloe vera to maintain smooth skin after you shave. Aloe vera is a natural ingredient that does not irritate the skin and provides fantastic lubrication so that your blade does not tug on the hairs as it cuts them. Your shaving experience will be a lot more pleasurable!

267. The sun can be a damaging force to skin. It produces ultraviolet rays that can cause damage to the skin. Wear a sunscreen lotion with an SPF of at least 15 and has the ability to block UVA and UVB rays. Apply to the skin before entering the sun (at least 20 minutes in advance).

268. Your skin care routine after age 50 should include exercises for the muscles in your face to combat sagging skin and wrinkles. To erase and prevent forehead wrinkles, raise your eyebrows while pulling down with two fingers placed above each eyebrow. Repeat 30 times, then relax. Do this two more times.

269. Keep your skin away from wet gloves and socks. Particularly in the winter months, these items can wreak havoc on your skin, causing itching, cracking and occasionally eczema. Resist the urge to put them on, and you will help your skin stay moist in the dry, cool weather.

270.   An important tip to consider when concerning acne is to be sure that you drink enough water. This is important because it is a healthy way to keep your skin from drying out. If you do not have enough water in your body to keep your skin moist then your body will produce more oil, increasing your chances of acne.

271.   Wearing sunscreen is one of the most important factors in having healthy skin. Sun exposure can cause freckles, wrinkles, sun spots and skin cancer. It can also make you look older. Sunscreen will help protect your skin against the harsh effects of the sun while giving you healthy, younger looking skin.

272.   If you are looking for improved results from exfoliation processes, extend the duration of your exfoliation treatments, not their intensity. Exfoliation should be a carefully-tuned treatment. Using abrasive products or aggressive scrubbing can harm your skin and counteract the benefits of exfoliation. Extending the length of your exfoliation process or repeating it can make it more effective without putting your skin at risk.

273.   As soon as you begin to notice the formation of red or purple stretch marks, consult your dermatologist about prescribing a topical tretinoin

preparation. These creams and lotions are the only effective treatment for stretch marks, but only when they are applied shortly after the initial appearance of the marks.

274.   Moisturizers are a good step in helping your skin stay healthy. Using a moisturizer after washing your face can give back the types of minerals that your skin needs to stay healthy. It is a good idea to make sure that your moisturizer is the right kind for your personal skin type or else you may end up just clogging your pores instead.

275.   To combat dry skin problems, eat more foods containing omega-3 fatty acids. Dry, scaly skin is sometimes a symptom of fatty acid deficiency, as these essential nutrients keep your skin moist. They also reduce inflammation which keeps blemishes from getting out of hand. Foods containing omega-3 fatty acids include walnuts, flax seeds, and fish like tuna and salmon.

276.   Strangely enough, you need to use moisturizer even if you have oily skin. If your skin is oily, and you skip the moisturizer, your skin will go into overtime producing oil to replace the oil you've just removed. So your face will end up oilier than before. Use a mild oil-free moisturizer so that your skin doesn't decide to rev up oil production again.

277.   Purchase products containing green tea extract to help maintain good skin. Green tea extract helps reduce unnecessary oils in your pores in addition to encouraging proper skin cell regeneration. A final benefit of green tea extract is that it is a natural product and may be best for those with extra sensitive skin.

278.   If you wear a lot of cosmetics, cleansing your face twice, can leave your skin clean and fresh. First, use a gentle cleanser that is specifically manufactured for cosmetic removal. After you rinse, follow up with a more soothing and hydrating cleanser, to make sure all residue from the makeup and previous cleanser are removed.

279.   Oatmeal is not just for breakfast. It helps itchy skin, too. Colloidal oatmeal can help with itchy skin caused by eczema, psoriasis, insect bites and poison ivy. Adding a cup or two of colloidal oatmeal to a warm bath helps treat itchy skin. Rinse with cool water after, and then pat dry with a towel. This can be done up to three times per day for relief.

280.   When you are putting on hand cream, don't forget to put a bit of lotion on your elbows. This easy step can help your elbows to look better and feel softer. A little bit of lotion goes a long way on

the elbows. Do not overlook this part of your body, because elbows need love, too.

281.   Start using anti-aging creams before wrinkles appear. Most anti-aging creams contain retinoids and Vitamin A, and applying these to your skin can not only reduce the signs of aging, they can delay their onset. Retinol can help skin to get rid of dead cells and increase the amount of collagen produced - leaving your face with a smooth, healthy glow.

282.   The smallest adjustments to your lifestyle can make a world of difference in protecting your skin from aging. For instance, you should switch to pillows made of satin instead of cotton. When you sleep at night, the cotton makes imprints on your face. Over time (think about it, you sleep every night!) these imprints can create permanent marks.

283.   To avoid redness and broken capillaries in your face, avoid exposing your skin to extreme heat. The heat causes increased blood flow to the peripheral areas in your body, which includes the skin of the face. The key areas to avoid are saunas and steam rooms, which get much warmer than any normal hot day.

284.   When you're in the shower washing your hair, it is easy to have the product drip down the side of

your face. Shampoos, conditioners and body washes contain harsh chemicals that may be damaging to your skin. To avoid harming your skin, try to lean your head back when you wash your hair and keep it away from your face as much as possible.

285.   You can give yourself a very beneficial facial massage. A facial massage helps your skin absorb moisturizers and oils much faster. Dispense a small amount of oil or moisturizer into your hands. Work your moisturizer or oil into your skin around your face in a circular motion, making sure to avoid the eyes.

286.   Even with sensitive skin - don't forget to tone. People with sensitive or dry skin are often advised not to use a toner, but this simply isn't the case. Choose an alcohol-free toner that is hypoallergenic. Use a cotton ball to apply the astringent to your face, and rather than rubbing, gently pat your face. This will help to get rid of any extra dirt and oil that your cleanser didn't remove.

287.   If you want to maintain soft, radiant skin, make sure that you use body wash in the shower. Body wash is a great alternative to soap, as it will not only soften your skin, but comes in a wide variety of aromas to improve your overall aura. Try to avoid body wash from touching your hair and face.

288.   If you need an exfoliate for your face and wish
to use an all natural method, try granulated sugar.
Granulated sugar, which is very inexpensive, or
sometimes free if acquired from restaurants, acts as
an abrasive when massaged into the skin. It
removes dead skin cells, allowing new skin cells to
surface.

289.   Touching your face with your bare hands is
poor skin care practice. Unless you just washed
them, your fingers are loaded with dirt and skin oil
that will transfer to your face. These contaminants
can block pores, cause infections and make any
existing skin conditions worse. Resist any and all
temptations to touch or rub your face.

290.   Clarify, heal and soothe your skin with a
nourishing mask made of honey and fresh apple.
Core and peel a small apple. Chop it and pulverize it
in your blender with one teaspoon of honey. Apply
the resulting mask to clean skin, and leave it on for
15 minutes. Rinse the mask off thoroughly using
warm water. Finish your beauty treatment with a
warm water rinse, a cold water rinse, and a splash of
toner.

291.   Make sure you drink plenty of water. Water is
beneficial to your body in many ways. It should be

no surprise that it also improves your complexion. Drinking water will help your skin get the moisture it requires. It will help your skin's elasticity as well as its general smoothness.

292.   Eating a healthy diet is a very important thing that you can do to take care of your skin. For example, eating foods that are rich in omega-3 fatty acids, such as salmon and avocados, can help decrease clogged pores, dry skin, and inflammation, and improve skin's youthfulness and elasticity.

293.   If you want to reduce unwanted redness in your skin, skip the store-bought products and try making your own redness reducer. That way you'll know exactly what's going on your skin, and you can avoid harsh ingredients that will potentially irritate your skin further or cause breakouts. You can make your skin treatment out of a little bit of jojoba oil and some Aloe Vera juice, both of which are gentle and readily available at the grocery or health food store.

294.   If your skin is oily, sensitive, or prone to breakouts, do away with bar soaps and bar cleansers. Instead, look for cleansers that are dispensed in pump or spray bottles. The moist, exposed surface of bar soaps, combined with the

humidity of an enclosed bathroom, encourages the growth of acne-causing bacteria.

295.   If you want to prevent wrinkles from forming on your face later in life, the best thing you can do is stay out of the sun. If you do have to go in the sun, always wear sunscreen with at least 25 SPF. If you can, try to wear a hat. By decreasing sun exposure, you lessen the damage it does to the elasticity of your skin.

296.   When you start to wear eye cream at night, be sure you know how to apply it properly. Do not roughly rub it on your skin. Instead, line a few dots of the cream under your eyes and on the eye lids. Gently pat the area around your eyes with the pads of your fingers until the cream blends in with your skin.

297.   If you have oily skin, then there are products out there for your specific skin type. You should opt for a gel cleanser to absorb oil and use a light moisturizer or serum with included sunscreen specifically labeled for oily skin. At any point in your day, you can also use oil blotting sheets to blot away excess oil to make your skin look and feel less oily.

298.   If one lives in a dry area or has skin that dries out during the drier times of the year such as winter in can be crucial for them to use a lotion. Using a lotion or moisturizer will keep ones skin from painful cracking as a result of being too dry.

299.   When you are putting on hand cream, don't forget to put a bit of lotion on your elbows. This easy step can help your elbows to look better and feel softer. A little bit of lotion goes a long way on the elbows. Do not overlook this part of your body, because elbows need love, too.

300.   Another great way to prevent your skin from looking dead and lifeless is to use tea tree oil to revitalize your skin. This fine natural product has been proven to prevent and treat a variety of skin problems. Tree tea oil is a great tool to get your skin on the right track today.

301.   Consult your doctor or dermatologist if you see big changes in the appearance of your skin or if you experience symptoms that do not get better. If you don't take your skin problems seriously, you can cause extreme damage to your skin, and quite possibly your health, by not seeking medical care.

302.   If you have been using a mister of water for your face, make sure to moisturize as well. The

water will evaporate on your skin which will dry it out. Moisturizing after words will prevent that from happening. You can also find misting products that also include moisturizers for a one stop solution.

303.   Consider cutting out high-glycemic foods in order to better care for your skin. Studies have shown that individuals who ate more protein and stayed away from foods like French fries and candy had better skin. In particular, they had significantly less pimples, indicating that what you eat has an impact on the way your skin looks.

304.   If conventional methods or natural methods of scar removal don't work for you, try dermabrasion. Dermabrasion involves taking away the top layers of skin to expose the younger skin underneath. Dermabrasion is done by using abrasive materials such as sandpaper or if you wish for a different solution, laser dermabrasion.

305.   The sun can be a damaging force to skin. It produces ultraviolet rays that can cause damage to the skin. Wear a sunscreen lotion with an SPF of at least 15 and has the ability to block UVA and UVB rays. Apply to the skin before entering the sun (at least 20 minutes in advance).

306.   Use a humidifier at home and at your work, if possible, to avoid dry skin. This helps to restore the moisture back to your skin. If your climate is a dry one, humidifiers can be a great help in preventing itchy, dry skin. Many affordable humidifiers are on the market today.

307.   To keep your skin looking good, you must learn how to wash properly. You don't want to use the wrong facial wash or scrub hard, because that can just irritate your skin. Find that right product for your skin type, rub in a circular manner and rinse well with warm water.

308.   If you have oily skin, make sure to use a gel based or foaming cleanser both in the morning and at night. Cleansers targeted specifically for your type of skin will help wash away excess oils and dirt clogging your pores. Make sure the product says it's for oily skin.

309.   When you are putting on hand cream, don't forget to put a bit of lotion on your elbows. This easy step can help your elbows to look better and feel softer. A little bit of lotion goes a long way on the elbows. Do not overlook this part of your body, because elbows need love, too.

310.   For healthy, good looking skin, avoid the tanning booth. People sometimes want to tan so they can look less than their years, but it can eventually do the opposite. Tanning creates premature aging and can damage the skin. A self-tanner will give you the same end result without the damage.

311.   One fantastic way to keep your skin looking healthy is to make sure that you do not use strong soaps. These strong soaps strip your skin of essential oils, causing your skin to look dry and dead. Instead, you should try to use more mild soaps, to keep your skin healthy longer.

312.   Do not forget to protect your lips with moisture too. Winter air can be very drying. Unless you take care to moisturize your lips with a lip balm, you will have the unpleasant experience of your lips becoming dry and cracked.

313.   Unfortunately, there is no permanent cure for those ugly bumps on the back of your legs known as cellulite. Unless you have amazing genes, every woman suffers from this problem. However, you can reduce their appearance on a day-to-day basis. Apply specialized cellulite creams that contain caffeine every morning. The caffeine in the lotion

will temporarily tighten the skin on your thighs, giving you smoothness that will last a few hours.

314.   If you would like the appearance of smoother, softer feet, then at bedtime, grab a bottle of olive oil from your kitchen cabinet and rub on a generous amount. Afterwards, throw on a pair of cotton socks on your feet and sleep with them on overnight. It may not be very attractive to wear cotton socks to bed, but you will reap the benefits with softer, smoother feet in the morning.

315.   If you want proper skin care then you have to make sure you don't smoke. Smoking contributes to wrinkles and reduces the amount of nutrients in your body that are helpful towards healthy skin, such as vitamin A. If you do happen to smoke and can't cut the habit then try your best to reduce the amount of smoke you consume, it would be better to quit altogether but any bit helps.

316.   One of the best things you can do to care for your skin, is to apply a lip balm with UV protection. Your lips contain extremely thin skin, which means they need extra protection from the sun. The use of lip balm will keep them from getting chapped and help prevent skin cancer from forming.

317.   Toner is one of the best things that you can use on your skin. A great toner will help to get rid of the impurities on your skin and even out the look of your face. Apply toner after you wash your face in the shower and follow with a top quality moisturizer with SPF.

318.   When cleansing your face, always remember to clean first with the cleanser of your choice and warm water. This cleansing process will open your pores and remove dirt and oil. Follow up your cleansing process with a cold water rinse to reduce pore size and refresh your skin. Finish up your routine with a toner to refine the pores and give your skin a glowing finish.

319.   Tanning causes skin cancer, liver spots, wrinkles and other damage to your skin. Whether you are tanning in the sun or in a tanning bed, your skin will suffer bad effects. If you must have a tan, get the spray-on kind; however, you will look far more attractive displaying the self-confidence to proudly wear the skin tone you already have!

320.   Applying your skin care products in order of their heaviness and density can help to give you the best absorption of those particular products. Start with the lightest of your products first and then continue on until you get to the heaviest of

products. This will allow you to get the full benefits of the lighter kinds of products without having the heavier ones drown them out.

321.   In order to keep your baby's skin healthy, you need to be able to treat diaper rash. This is important because if left unattended, this will be extremely painful and may become infected. To treat diaper rash you need to remove diaper, expose the area to open air, wash with a warm cloth and apply diaper rash cream.

322.   For shaving legs, underarms, or beard, be sure to use a mild, low pH, moisturizing soap and lather well. This will help lubricate the skin so that your razor blade glides over it harmlessly. Look for products created especially for sensitive skin. Alternately, use a very mild hair conditioner with a few drops of sunflower or peanut oil added for pain-free shaving.

323.   If you have an excess amount of oil or sebum on your skin, try to use oil absorbing sheets periodically, during the day. These sheets can help to control the oil that your body produces and limit the effect that it has on your skin. Oil helps trap bacteria, so the less oil on your skin, the better.

324.   If you have excessively dry skin, you must apply your moisturizer many times throughout the day. It is especially important to apply moisturizer after washing your hands; many people find that it is easier to remember to moisturize when they have a separate bottle in their desk, nightstand, or vehicle. Reapplying moisturizer allows the skin to fully absorb and use the nutrients in the product.

325.   If you have sensitive skin, be careful when trying out new products. No matter what skin type you do have, sensitivity can also be a factor. Pay attention when buying skin care products, and check labels to make sure there's no ingredients that you know aggravate your skin. If you're not sure, buy products specifically designed for sensitive skin.

326.   A simple tissue can tell you what type of skin you have. If you are unsure of your skin type, take a tissue, unfold it, and press it to your face. If you see oil on the tissue in the areas of the forehead, nose, and cheeks - you have oily skin. If it only shows oil on the forehead and nose, you have combination skin. No oil means you have normal or dry skin. If your skin feels taught, it is likely on the dry side.

327.   To keep your lips looking smooth and luscious, make sure to wear a lip gloss or lipstick that has sunscreen in it. Just as the sun can damage the rest

of your skin, it can also damage your lips, leaving them dried and cracking. Wearing a lip gloss with sunscreen can help protect your lips from the sun's damaging rays.

328.   The first step in fixing your skin problems is figuring out what type of skin you have. Find out what your skin type is so that you can get a product that will help your issues. Determine your skin type before you waste money on ineffective regimens.

329.   To avoid getting wrinkles and worn looking skin, wear skin protection while in direct sunlight. Types of protection include sunscreen, hats, and clothes such as long sleeve shirts, pants and skirts. The UV rays in sunlight can cause severe damage to skin, blemishes, dry skin, sun burn and cancer.

330.   To improve your complexion right away, you should exfoliate your skin. Exfoliating removes dead and dull skin cells, making your skin looking healthy and bright. A gentle exfoliating scrub can revitalize your skin without damaging it. Regular exfoliation can reduce the visibility of scars and wrinkles, and can also lead to fewer breakouts.

331.   One way to take care of your skin is to exfoliate longer. If you are aiming to deeply exfoliate, do not try to scrub harder as you clean your skin. Simply

wipe longer because using too much pressure can actually be harmful to your skin, negating the beneficial effects of the product.

332.   Get plenty of exercise. Exercising frequently helps your skin maintain a healthy fresh glow by regulating the oxygen flow in your body. Make sure you avoid wearing makeup while you exercise because your it can trap your sweat within your pores and cause a breakout. Take a clean cloth with you to wipe your face every time you sweat to avoid any dirt clogging your pores.

333.   Hyaluronic acid is a very powerful skin hydrating serum. If your skin is feeling very dry beyond repair, buy some hyaluronic acid and apply to the afflicted areas with a dropper. This acid has the most moisturizing and hydrating effects on the market today. It is able to hold up to 1000 times its weight in water.

334.   If you wear a lot of makeup then you need to use a lot of cleanser. Cleaning your face twice after a heavy makeup day will cleanse and protect your skin from the effects. Try using a gentle cleanser that is designed for makeup removal first and then follow up with your regular routine.

335.   To have glowing skin, it is imperative that you get your full six to eight hours of sleep every single night. While you are asleep, that's when your skin cells work to repair your skin. Not getting enough rest will interrupt your re-growth and it will show up on your face the next day.

336.   Sunless tanner is a great way to have a safe glow all year round. However, these products can sometimes cause breakouts. In order to prevent breakouts from self tanning products, read the label carefully, and make sure it contains the word "non comedogenic." That is a scientific term that means the product will not clog your pores. Thus, breakouts will be eliminated.

337.   Be sure to use plenty of the right kind of sunscreen before going outside if you want to take proper care of your skin. Put it on a half hour before you go outside and reapply it every two hours. If you sweat heavily or get wet, you should reapply it more frequently.

338.   Vitamin E is an important vitamin to help you improve the look of your hair and skin. Vitamin E is rich in antioxidants and is able to fight off free radicals. There are numerous foods which are rich in vitamin E, including papaya, blueberries and

almonds. Also there is vitamin A in darker, leafy greens.